Dear Friend

Dear Friend

Letters of Encouragement, Humor, and
Love for Women with Breast Cancer

Gina L. Mulligan

GIRLS LOVE MAIL

CHRONICLE BOOKS
SAN FRANCISCO

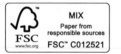

Library of Congress Cataloging-in-Publication Data available.

ISBN 978-1-4521-6342-0

Manufactured in China

MIX
Paper from
responsible sources
FSC
www.fsc.org
FSC™ C012521

Art direction by Vanessa Dina
Design by Lizzie Vaughan

10 9 8 7 6 5 4 3 2 1

Chronicle Books LLC
680 Second Street
San Francisco, California 94107
www.chroniclebooks.com

FOR MY FRIEND:

THIS BOOK IS FOR

the women who fight;
the families and friends
who hold steady;
the coworkers who listen;
the volunteers who raise
money and awareness;
the health professionals
who won't give up; and
those who came before.

With grace, resilience,
and courage we triumph.

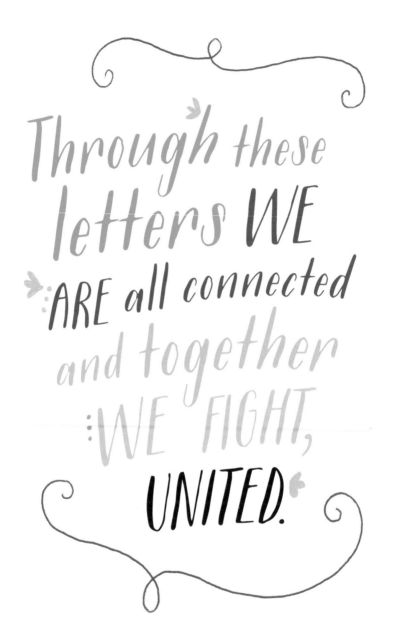

❯··· Friends in Spirit ···❮

DEAR FRIEND,

Letters are sacred mementos we lovingly save in decorative boxes, memories captured to relive again and again. Yet the gentle beauty of a handwritten letter seems largely forgotten in our age of text messages and emails. After working for five years on a novel comprised entirely of letters, I felt connected to what I consider the lost art of letter writing. However, not until I was diagnosed with breast cancer did I understand that a few words on paper are more than a keepsake. A handwritten letter is a gift with the ultimate power to heal and inspire.

Hearing I had cancer was a frightening shock, but what happened in the following weeks changed my perspective on kindness: I began receiving letters and cards from friends of friends, strangers. People I'd never met took time to tell me I was a hero, a warrior, a survivor. Their support filled me with hope and reminded me that I wasn't alone.

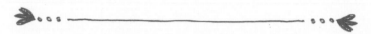

Once I beat cancer, I knew what I had to do.

In August 2011, I set out with the mission of getting handwritten letters of encouragement to women newly diagnosed with breast cancer. My husband and I wrote letters at our kitchen table, and then we roped in family and friends to help. We donated the letters to breast cancer centers who gave them to their patients. As we shared our message, people responded. Hundreds, then thousands of letters began coming in from around the country and then from around the world. By simply asking, caring individuals of all ages and backgrounds wrote heartfelt, beautiful words to encourage you, their friend in spirit.

The idea for this collection began when an extraordinary letter again touched my life. On simple white stationery was a note from an oncology nurse. For over twenty years, she'd cared for women with breast cancer and now she was a patient in her own clinic. Rather than focus on the irony or injustice, she wanted nothing more than to use her diagnosis to make her an even better caretaker. Not only could she answer her patients' medical questions, but now, for the first time, she *experienced* their distress.

She felt "blessed" for her understanding, and even while undergoing her own arduous chemotherapy, she set aside time to visit patients, the women she called "sisters." The best in humanity can't be ignored. There was more we could do.

The letters in this book were written by survivors and their family members, friends, colleagues, and others wanting to encourage you, a breast cancer warrior. Some of the letters are profound, as letter writers share their personal struggles and heartaches in order to express deep appreciation for your journey. Others are lighthearted and fun so you can take a breath or set aside your cares for a few moments. There are even funny letters to make you laugh. Laughter is fine medicine, indeed.

Even though we live in a fast-paced society, I hope these words lift your spirits, help you heal, and remind you that you're never alone. Through these handwritten letters, we are all connected and together we fight, united.

Gina L. Mulligan

FOUNDER OF GIRLS LOVE MAIL

Dear Friend –

Know that there are many of us out here who care that you are experiencing this difficulty. My thoughts: Be crazy. Be funny. Be silly. Be weird. Be whatever you would like to be. Because life is unpredictable to be anything but happy. Try to be that strong, brave woman we all know you are. Put your flip-flops on and go to where you're happy. Take those who love you with to share your joy or struggles. Take care –

Barb

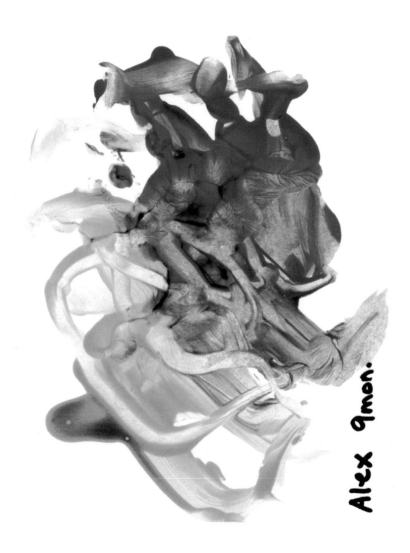

Alex 9mon.

Dear Friends,

I know, and have known women who have been diagnosed with breast cancer. Some of these diagnoses were for 'later stage' breast cancer – some were for 'early stage' breast cancer. Nevertheless, when that phone call comes in from your doctor saying you have breast cancer – at that point, all your focus is "you have breast cancer" and it doesn't really matter if its 'late stage' or 'early stage'. The words "breast cancer" is devastating!! I am aware of your fears and anxiety; I have felt these words too.

The road ahead might be long, but with the love and support from friends and family you will come out of this. There have been so many recent developments in breast cancer research and treatment, that when your treatment is complete you will be able to celebrate life to the fullest!!

Keep positive thoughts — I have, and now I'm proud to say, I have been a breast cancer survivor for almost 22 years!!

Know that you are loved)

Pearl :)

Dear friend,

I am so happy, the wig that has been on my head for over 1 year has been put to rest! I had long straight blonde hair, now I have short, curly salt and pepper hair (I dyed it last week)

and I love it!!,
I hope the curls
stay, so easy to
take care of and I
deserve that, see
we have to look
at the positive!

Stay Strong
And positive

"Your friend
in Brst Cancer

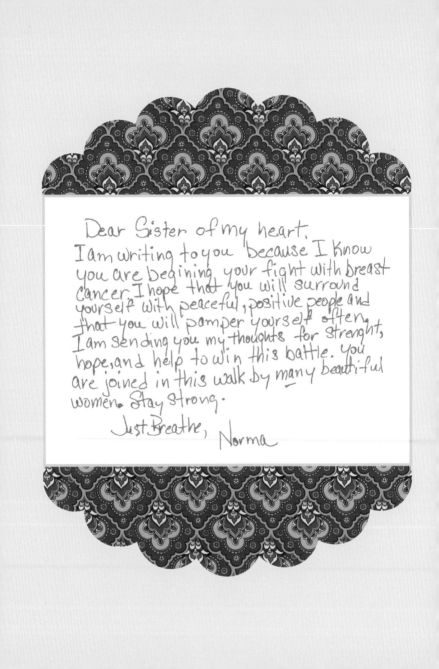

Dear Sister of my heart,
I am writing to you because I know
you are begining your fight with breast
cancer. I hope that you will surround
yourself with peaceful, positive people and
that you will pamper yourself often.
I am sending you my thoughts for strenght,
hope, and help to win this battle. You
are joined in this walk by many beautiful
women. Stay strong.

Just Breathe,
Norma

My Dear Sister,

Just as you probably remember where you were, how you felt, and perhaps even what you were wearing on 9/11/01, so too will you always vividly recall every detail of the day and way you received your Cancer Diagnosis. As you begin your unique Journey through the Cancer Maze, scared - as we all are - I'll be virtually holding your hand. When you finally reach and walk through the Maze's Exit, I'll be there in Spirit to say, "Welcome to the Survivors' Sorority!"

♡ Stephanie the Survivor

Dear Sister,

As you read this you may be feeling overwhelmed and sad OR you might be having a great day and seeing beauty everywhere. A breast cancer adventure is just that - an adventure. It's got highs and lows. I do hope that knowing someone is sending you positive thoughts helps alleviate any stress. I was diagnosed at 35 with triple negative breast cancer. I just celebrated my 36th birthday yesterday. I am so grateful for everything I have learned and for all the little things that are so beautiful like the rain, clouds, breeze, frozen yogurt, ☺ and of course smiles!

May your life be filled with smiles!

— Larissa R

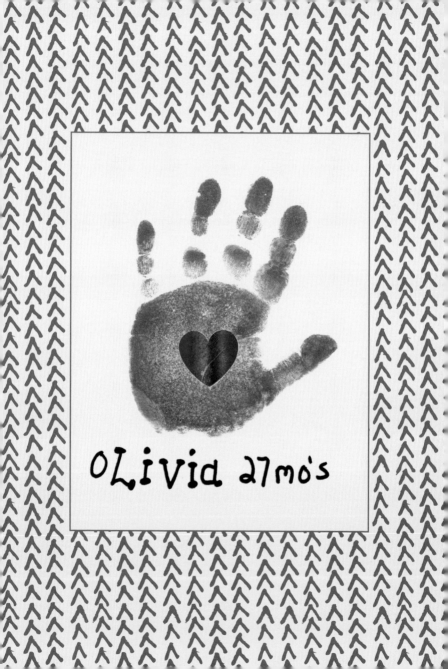

OLiViA 27mo's

Dear Fellow Survivor,

Cancer made me a better mother. It made me
cherish every moment of my boys' lives. It made
me not want to miss any of their school activities,
baseball games, cub scouts, etc. I was diagnosed
with breast cancer when my sons were 1 and 3
years old.

Cancer made me a better wife. It made me
appreciate my husband more. It made me not
waste so much time arguing about the small
stuff. I was diagnosed with cancer when my
husband and I were married 7 years.

Cancer made me a better daughter. It made
me visit with my parents more. It made me
call them just to say hi. I was 28 years

old when the doctor told me I had breast cancer. My parents were with me.

Cancer made me a better teacher. When I was diagnosed, I had been teaching elementary school for 5 years.

Cancer made me a better friend. I love to laugh with my girlfriends. When I had my mastectomy, some of my friendships were very new.

My sons are now 25 and 27 years old.

My husband + I have been married for 31 years.

I have been a daughter for 52 years. →

This will be my 30th year teaching.

My "new" friendships are 20+ years and counting!

Cancer made me better. It made me stronger. This may sound strange, but I'm glad I had cancer. I think I beat it and you can, too!

I'm writing to you today because cancer made you better already. It made you stronger. You have gotten through the hardest thing that you have ever, ever had to do.

You WILL be o.k. You will survive! One day, you will write a letter like this

to another woman. You will tell her
that many, many years ago, you were
scared too. You will tell her she will
get through chemo and radiation and
whatever else she chooses to do.

You will hear the word CANCER one
day in the future and you will think, oh
yeah, I had that once many, many years
ago...

I wish you happiness and love with
your family and friends. Most of all,
I wish you a very long and peaceful
life. Cancer has ended all over you...

You have just begun!!!
Sincerely, Cindy L.

Dear Sister,
Today I want you to know that you are LOVED. There is a circle of women who are surrounding you to offer you strength and support. We love you and are sending you supportive

thoughts and hugs.
You are a strong
warrior and you
are never alone.
The fellowship of
women is with
you.
Peace and love,
Karen B.

Dear Friend,

I am thinking of you and wishing you sunny days. I know, for a fact, that there is "light at the end of the tunnel." I was a recent widow when I was diagnosed with cancer. I thought my life was over. My family was very supportive but it was through the wonderful and caring efforts of my "old retired teacher girlfriends" that made me survive. They just would not let me give up. Their calls, visits, gifts and prayers gave me the boost that I needed.

Now that I am healthy I try to pay forward some of the love I was shone. May some of that love come to you, and when you are well, may you "give back".

A funny aside! When my hair started to fall out I would shake my towel out my bedroom window. The next spring my little neighbor joyfully brought me a birdsnest. He said, "Look how soft it is!" It was MY hair! Is that the ultimate in recycling?

May you find many occasions to smile.

Peace,
Maddy O.

Dear Friend,

This little note is filled with many good wishes for you. A wish for _peace_ to calm your heart, _love_ to see you through, and _strength_ for your fight and your healing.

When you need extra encouragement, remember that your "sisters" everywhere are thinking of you and sending their positive thoughts. You are special and you are loved! Sending a hug, Amy

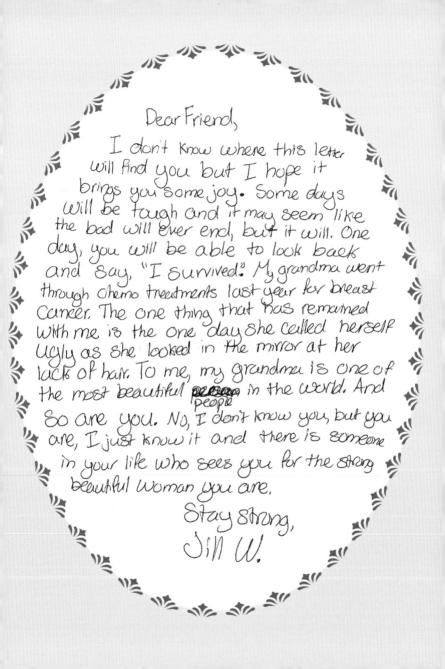

Dear Friend,

I don't know where this letter will find you but I hope it brings you some joy. Some days will be tough and it may seem like the bad will ever end, but it will. One day, you will be able to look back and say, "I survived." My grandma went through chemo treatments last year for breast cancer. The one thing that has remained with me is the one day she called herself ugly as she looked in the mirror at her lack of hair. To me, my grandma is one of the most beautiful ~~person~~ people in the world. And so are you. No, I don't know you, but you are, I just know it and there is someone in your life who sees you for the strong beautiful woman you are.

Stay strong,

Jill W.

Dear Friend,

Although our cancers are different ~ mine is ovarian ~ we probably share many of the same thoughts & feelings.

As you adjust to your diagnosis, you will be amazed by your strength. Sometimes we don't know how strong we are until we find ourselves in a difficult situation.

However, don't be afraid to lean on others as you go through this. That can be hard for those of us who are used to putting others before ourselves. Now is the time to put yourself first.

My thoughts & prayers are with you & I send my very best wishes for a speedy & complete recovery.

Hugs,
Joyce M.

Jimmy

Hello my name is Jimmy. I am nine and
to pray for your happiness, I am six years
old. I have a good school my teacher
Mrs. Dunbar is very nice maybe if you met
her you would see. My dog org. Cant hear.
Lukky and Wink my dog is blind in one
eye he was born like that my dog has the
hair color of gold Wink and Luke are
nice. The PE teacher is nice to in my
school. One time we played a game with
red ball and a blue ball and the red ball was the
tagging ball and the blue ball is the untagging
ball.

Dear Friend,

Since you are receiving this, I hope it shows
you have support and are even from people
you do not know. My mother fought breast
cancer over twenty-five years ago, and her
humor and drive carried her through some
dark moments. I'm proud to say she is
turning 70 this year, still going strong and
still driving a Corvette because it is "a practical car."

She lives on the ocean. The ocean has salt spray. Salt spray causes rust on anything but a fiberglass car. Therefore, a Corvette is only practical.

I never thought mail from an anonymous person would help, but when I was deployed recently to Afghanistan, it did my heart good to hear from people everywhere. I hope this does the same for you, and know that you are in good company with 70-year-old Corvette-driving seniors.

Yours,

Scott Y.

Dear friend,
   I wrote a poem
         for you—
   Lighthouse,
   Cancer warrior—
   Symbols of strength.

   Storms crash
   around them
   But they are
   Strong
   And endure.
   Beacons of light,
   Beacons of hope
   Standing fearless
   In the dark of
   Night.
                DONNA K

Dearest Lovely Lady,
I wrote a poem for you:

Sit outside in your favorite place,
To the rising sun raise your
    beautiful face.
Take a deep breath and close your
    gorgeous eyes,
Breathe out, relax your body with
    a long deep sigh.

With eyes still closed listen to every
    sound,
Wind chimes dancing, birds singing
    nature all around,
With both arms hug yourself really
    tight.
Know that in your world at this
moment all is right.

At day's end return to your special
    place.
Look to the starry sky and
    recognize a familiar face.
Count each and every star in the
    sky so blue
For every star represents good wishes
    and love sent especially for you.

Best Wishes
    Thinking of You!!
        JEllen B.

Dear Friend,

I watched my sister-in-law go through breast cancer. She was a pillar of strength throughout the whole ordeal. After her mastectomy, she decided to knit herself some "boobies" to use in her new bra. She was funny and silly, knitting "boobies" in all kinds of colors, stripes, polka dots, some even looked like fruit! It made us all laugh which made us realize that she really was ok - emotionally!

Sometimes a little laugh goes a long way to raise a persons spirit. My thoughts are with you.

Love,

Ricki B.

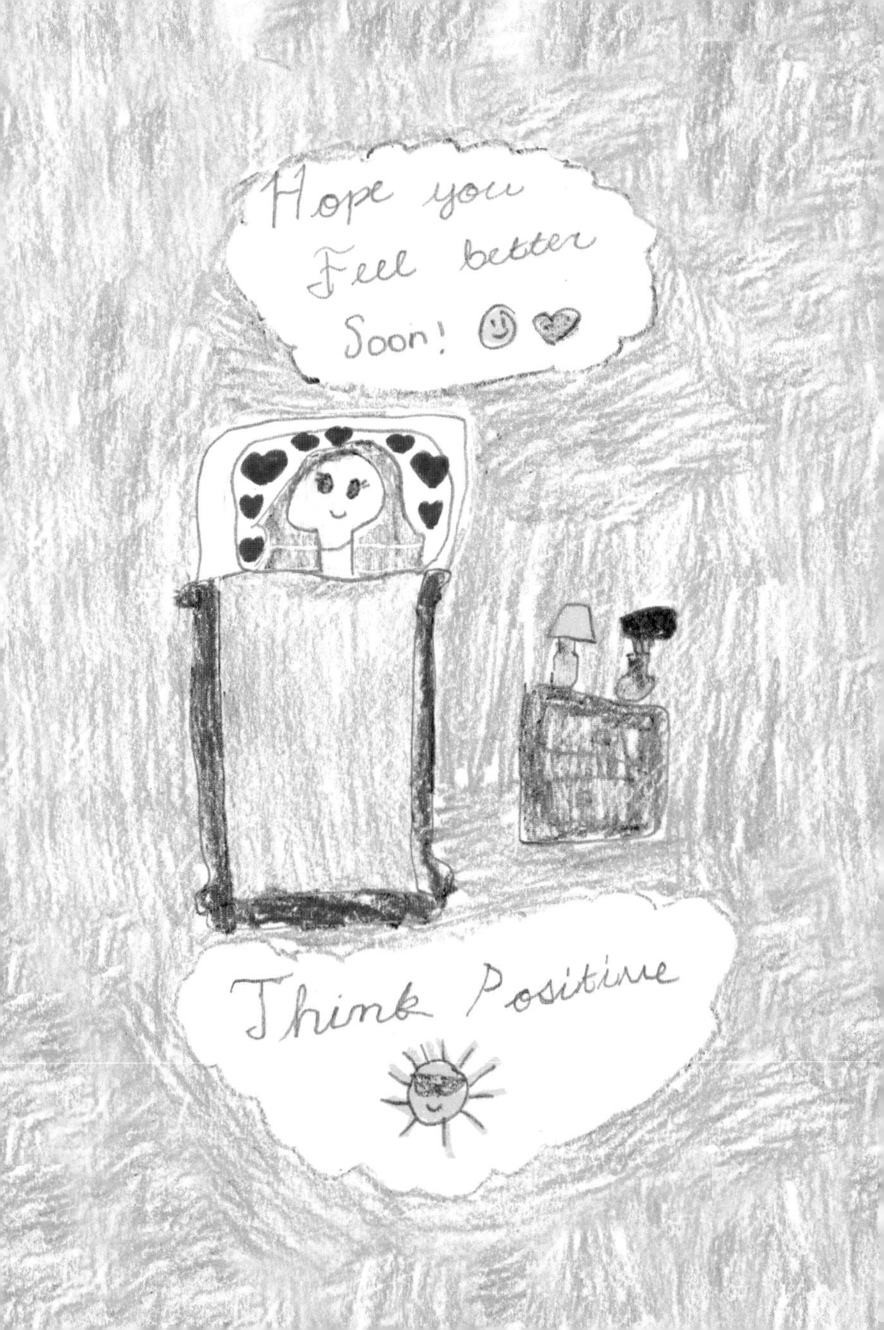
Hope you
Feel better
Soon!
Think Positive

Dear Sister,

Four years after my own diagnosis of breast cancer, I'm thinking of you and wishing you peace at this difficult, disorienting time.

I hope you have already discovered there is tremendous love and support around you, even from strangers. All survivors and you are one, already — are your family and we will provide warm well of support to you through the years whenever you need it.

I wish you all the courage you need in dealing with this illness. Even when cancer seems to dominate everything, there are moments, precious moments, you can enjoy. Being with loved ones, in nature, whatever makes you laugh — these things cancer cannot take from you.

Right now I see close my eyes and imagine you four years from now as I am — feeling great, having just walked 3 miles on a beautiful beach, grateful. Love, Ann B.

Dear amazing woman —

Here I sit on a Sunday afternoon with a group of amazing women — and a few amazing guys too — making cards of love, encouragement and support for women like you. We want to do everything we can to offer you what you need on your journey. May this be a wishing card — Whatever you are hoping for, wish on this card and our good vibes will be with you. Our circle of love will support you and your family. All the best wishes! Peace + love, Amy

Dear Friend,

My name is Hannah and I want to congradulate you on your success so far! I realize that this is a difficult journey for you, but I know that you are handling it marvelously. Being Courageous can be as simple as waking up in the morning — which you must have done to be reading this! See, you are braver than you thought.

Anyone who has the will to survive a life threatening illness is a hero in my book. As you continue your battle, know that there are people who support you and wish the best for you. Even the personally unafflicted feel the suffering caused by this disease and we all fight to put an end to it. You are never alone.

Sincerely, Hannah

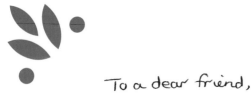

To a dear friend,

You may be a long way away
from me but I wanted to connect
with you today and to say you are
loved, you are special and you have
my support. I want you to be you,
smile when you can and don't lose yourself
and your uniqueness that makes you who
you are. My hopes and wishes are with
you, truly and from my heart and every part
of me. I am sending you my strength and
positivity, my strength and determination
and hope that it makes a difference to you.

You are an amazing woman and I hope
that my letter makes your day a little
brighter and easier to bear.

Be safe, be strong,
much love,

Soulla C.

x x x   x x x

Dear Sister,

My Mother was diagnosed with Breast cancer when I was I. I know how you would feel well not really but I know its really hard. I think I waandt to get up a Breast Cancer writing club.

My MoM is still ok and I'm sure you will too. Im close to be 10, I'm in 4th grade. Do you have any kids. Can I tell you something that I got for Chris-tmas, I Hope you like taylor swist because I got tickers. My Family and Friends will storm you with prayers.

Thank you.

Matathea M

Dear Sister,

Hello, my dear sister! How I wish I could join you for a Kitchen table Chats! I'll bring your favorite coffee, tea, or soda and we'll sit for hours, sharing to our heart's content.

You have many people wishing you well right now. More than you know. We're wishing you the best that life has to offer. What would that look like for you?

Wouldn't it make Spring tulips and trips to the river to call at spoonfuls of relaxation in TLC? Afternoons of gas to that Pip! and long drives Spring cleaning? or stretches of relaxation in planting Christmas and sunny spring summers at (suggest!) mean, it all it?

that would you rake leaves and fall back on them, looking up at the clouds to see the shapes they resemble? Or sit by our favorite books or movies. Maybe share hot chocolate and could share take an afternoon to the quiet pleasure of coloring the straw-light of in order to log the the colors God cherishes the experience by your favorite pet. breathing their the sound of their spirit hope you spend garage every dog joined free page join the God spirit.

Love,
Carmen

Dear Friend,

My name is Jadon. I am a student in Tampa.
       Though I'm sure I can't imagine what you're
going through, I just wanted to let you know that we
are all thinking of you. You can beat this, I know
you can! Stay strong and remember that you're never
alone. I know what it's like to be sick, though it
be a different kind. I had a severe curvature in my
spine and needed major surgery to correct it; the
recovery took almost 2 years. I know what it's like
to feel helpless. Always remember to stay strong!
Time heals, and things can get better if you fight with
all your strength.
       Sincerely, Jadon

Hi friend,

I grew up with the saying women
were the weaker sex. What a crazy idea!
We are very strong; we care for children,
husbands, friends and neighbors, putting others
first. Now my strong brave lady, it is time
to put yourself first. All your strength &
energy need to focus on you, getting you
well. And you will get well. I'm living
proof. I was diagnosed with ovarian cancer
in 1995 and I'M here to provide others
hope. Believe in your body ability to heal
itself and it will. Faith can move mountains.

Linda B.

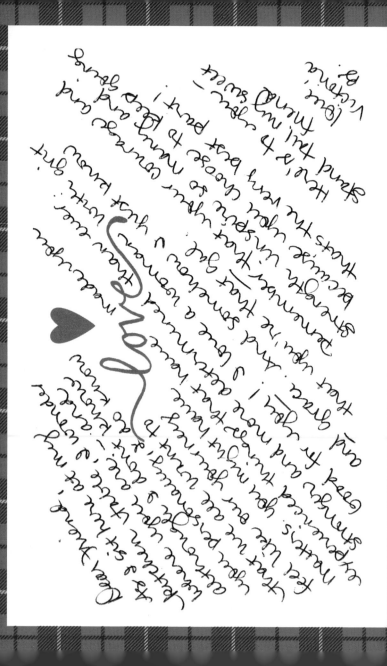

Friend —

I've always liked the French translation of our English word:

"Survival" ←

In English, it almost feels like it means just barely getting by, or through something, etc.

In French, the word is written: ↓

"Survivre"

which, when it is literally broken down, looks like:

"Sur | vivre"
ON   TO LIVE

I think to fight
to just barely
eek by feels so
much more
frustrating to fight.
But - to fight to
go "on to live"
makes the stakes
even higher &
a more ferocious
fighter somehow.

My wish for you:
... may your fight
be ferocious and
then - on to 'live'.

a wish for you:
Survive

Sincerely-
aM

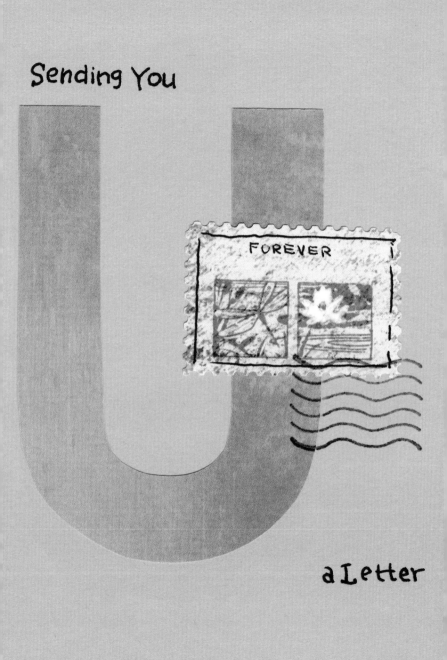

To a fighter,

Until now, you had other
places to be

Until now, you had better
things to do

Until now, you didn't take
time to think

Until now, you hadn't
really planned

Until now, you might have
missed rainbows

Until now, you could
have skipped
goodnight kisses

Until now, you didn't
   take time for you
Until now, you hadn't
   counted your friends
recently

Now, you appreciate
   each day, each
   friend, each ex-
   perience as you
   work toward THEN

Until then,
   know that I care

Sandy

Dear friend,

I am thinking of you and all that you have gone though. You have my support and my admiration.

My mother had breast cancer. I cried many tears but she didn't! She had a great confidence and she beat it. I want to encourage you to be positive and know that I am cheering you on to a complete recovery.

I know you have had tough days. May you have a strong resolve to continue your bravery. You are my "heroine".

Remember, I am on your side and will continue to think of you and your progress.

With friendship,
Sharon Z.

Let me
hear your
battle cry!!

Dear friend,

I cannot even begin to comprehend the emotions going through your head. I wish I could. Life would be far easier if empathy was, too. But I can only try.

In August of 2015, I began my freshman year in High School. I had just left a ten-year dance career, which I had been so firmly invested in, I hadn't tried much of anything else. Per my parents' recommendation, along with theatre classes, I signed up for journalism.

The day I met my teacher, I was still extremely shy and rather terrified, and she overwhelmed me with her polar personality. I was suddenly thrown headfirst into a class where critique was frequent, but not unkind; where students were treated with the kindness and encouragement one would give an equal; a place where I was not the best, but was not the worst, either.

Somehow, with her huge, bubbly personality, my teacher convinced me to join a series of competitions. At my second, I won first place. Again at the third. I began climbing the ranks, finding more and more competition, until finally, thanks to the endless encouragement my teacher gave me, I not only won first in my state, but found my home in life - writing for newspapers.

And in the midst of all of this, my teacher had breast cancer.

She missed most of our first semester due to treatment. We mostly conversed via email. She graded countless papers from her hospital bed, never delaying in her grading and assigning new projects. Despite the challenges of cancer, she continued to push her classes to success.

That is what I wish for you. Cancer presents tons of obstacles, and they may seem unbeatable, but a disease does not have to destroy who you are and what you stand for. Know that behind the writing of this note is a girl who supports you along with countless others, but not just because you got a disease; more because you still have the power to influence others despite it. You have cancer, yes, but that does not define you; don't let it.

Sincerly,
Erin S.
Grade 10

Dear friend,

I'm thinking of you; though we don't know each other, we have something in common, — breast cancer.

If I tell you a little about my experience, I hope it will help you to have hope...

My breast cancer was diagnosed in June of 1999; almost 15 years ago... I had a lumpectomy, radiation, chemo therapy, and ten years of tamoxifen; and I'm happy to say I'm a survivor, at age 83.

During those years we kept busy, and our only two grandchildren (boys, now age 6 and 3½) arrived...

I tried to get as much rest as I could, especially at the beginning, and learned to accept help, whenever friends asked, and treated myself to small fun treats, to have thing to look forward to. One of my favorite thoughts was - and still is - from The Little Engine That Could; - "I think I can. I think I can." which is now - "I thought I could, I thought I could". I wish for you - hope and strength and peace.

Anne Z.

Beautiful,

Strength.

Beauty. Sister.

Hope. love.

faith. Cancer.

These words are often used to describe breast cancer, or the cancer patient, but what do these words really mean?

Strength: quality of state or being. Something you are chalk-ful of!

Beauty: a quality in a person that gives intence pleasure to the mind. Might be the best descriptive word to describe you.

Hope: an emotional state that promotes belief in the positive. What I have in you.

Sister: a girl in relation to others.

love: an intence feeling of deep affection

faith: complete trust in someone or something. I have faith you can beat this.

Cancer: a disese caused by an uncontrolable division of cells in the body. It doesnt define you

Deryn Y.

Dear Sister,

I'm writing to support + encourage you at a time that is so challenging + difficult. It is an honor to be able to reach out, and though we will probably never meet, please know that there are many of us out here who are joined with you in your struggle. I had a diagnosis of an aggressive form of breast cancer eight years ago, and I'm so grateful, now, for every minute of my life.

At the time – and for months – I tried to do everything I could to keep my spirits up, to remain optimistic + hopeful. In my fear, I also tried to do whatever I could to participate in decision-making. Some days, I felt so down + hopeless. Fortunately, I was able to work part-time, so I could get treatments but also have hours each day where I couldn't just dwell on my illness. Because, mostly, that's about all that I did.

I was ~~sure~~ shocked when I was diagnosed. I still can see exactly where I was standing when I got that phone call. Then, I was a nervous wreck for a few months. Once my treatment plan was in place, I felt a bit relieved—like, at least, there was some hope + attempt to help me.

We live in a city where there are many medical centers, so I tried to "research" what hospital would be the "best." So, in looking back, for many months, I drove myself crazy—always second-guessing doctors—I was almost too many choices—I was terrified that I wouldn't pick the BEST one.

Finally, with support from friends and family, I learned to "let go," to trust my doctors. And they were great. I still check-in yearly, and I realize now that they were always wonderful; I was too scared, at the time, to understand that.

→ over

Emotionally, I didn't do so well. I couldn't conjure up the serenity + optimism that others seemed to have in the face of cancer. I felt like I wasn't processing my experience "correctly."

Because I was still working, I worried that I wasn't having a "life-changing" (in a good way) experience - something I'd heard others talk about. There were no local support groups that I could attend while working (we were 1-2 hrs from the city, and the only excellent support group took place during my work day.) It took me a couple of years to realize that my outlook on life had/has changed as a result of my experience → and that my appreciation of small + big things has expanded.

I'll share one piece of advice given to me by a friend who'd also had breast cancer. When I was tiring of talking about it with people (mostly kind co-workers who were trying to be supportive,) my friend said that I didn't always need to engage in that conversation. Sometimes I just didn't have the emotional energy to tell my story. I learned that I could say that, politely, to people while expressing my appreciation for their concern. Everyone totally understood!

I hope that this helps - a little. You are not alone. Please know that whatever you are feeling - both the ups + the downs, has been shared or is being shared by many of us. One day at a time was a helpful reminder to me. Let people love to help you. Do your research (not on the internet at midnight - too scary,) ask questions (of your doctors, talk to family + trusted friends, ask questions (of your doctors too!). If there's a local support group that you feel is helpful - give it a chance. Know that you are stronger than you may realize right now.

I know that there have been big advances in treatment options over the last few years - try to stay hopeful. Love yourself + let others love you.

All my best - my unknown friend ♡

Cynthia

You
Will
Be
OK

Dear friend,

When I was diagnosed with bladder cancer I was shocked I was 54 years old and had so much to do. I got depressed and wasn't doing anything but feeling sorry for myself. My sister gave me this poem.

"When we wake up in the morning, we have two simple choices. Go back to bed and dream, or wake up and chase those dreams."

I choose to chase my dreams. Now I'm so busy with family and friends I don't have time to think about my cancer.

I wish you the best of days ahead. Love of friends
Tammy S.

Dear Friend,
    My name is maddie and I
wanted to tell you how strong &
brave you are. Your also not
alone on your fight with cancer. About
7 years ago, my mom had breast
cancer. We caught it very late & nobody
thought she was going to live. But
guess what, she did. The love and
support people gave us was invincable
to her desiese. She beat it, and is as
healthy as ever today. I believe the
same will happen to you. You are
sostrong and I think with love &
support, you will surley beat cancer.
If you ever feel alone, just think that
people love you, and truely care about
you. And always remember, that
no cancer can stand up to the
power of love.
        Sincerely,
            maddie

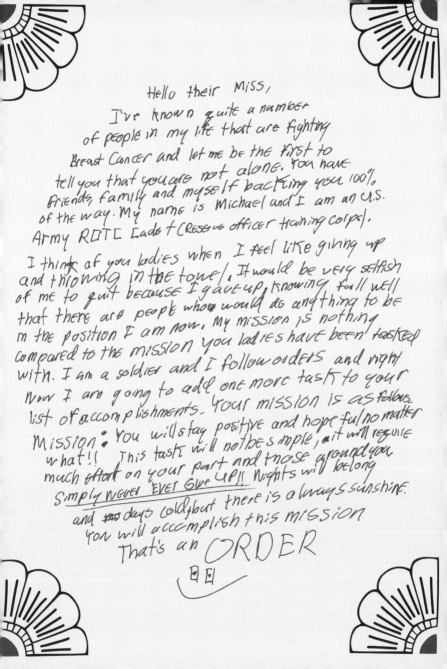

Hello their Miss,

I've known quite a number of people in my life that are fighting Breast Cancer and let me be the first to tell you that you are not alone. You have friends, family and myself backing you 100% of the way. My name is Michael and I am an U.S. Army ROTC Cadet (Reserve officer training corps).

I think of you ladies when I feel like giving up and throwing in the towel. It would be very selfish of me to quit because I gave up, knowing full well that there are people who would do anything to be in the position I am now. My mission is nothing compared to the mission you ladies have been tasked with. I am a soldier and I follow orders and right now I am going to add one more task to your list of accomplishments. Your mission is as follows.

Mission: You will stay positive and hopeful no matter what!! This task will not be simple, it will require much effort on your part and those around you. Simply never EVER Give UP!! Nights will belong and days cold, but there is always sunshine. You will accomplish this mission

That's an ORDER

Dear Friend,

Last night I was in charge of Science Night at my son's elementary school. We had parents and community members who work in the sciences set up tables all over the cafeteria with science-related activities. A NASA scientist brought a vacuum chamber and let the kids help him experiment by putting different things in it, sucking out the air, and seeing what happened. Torturing Marshmallow Peeps in it was especially fun for the students.

oh no!

VERY BADLY DRAWN MARSHMALLOW PEEPS AWAIT THEIR TURN IN THE VACUUM CHAMBER

And did you know that a can of Diet Coke will float in a tank of water, but a can of Dr. Pepper will sink? (It's the corn syrup.) Who could have guessed it?

All over the school cafeteria, kids learned about weather, dentistry, snakes (they even got to hold one), planets, butterflies, static electricity, and more. We gave away a lot of free science-related books, and everyone got to eat pizza. The kids had a blast! And I think they learned a lot, too.

Sssss... where's MY pizzza?

I'm telling you all this to let you know that I'm trying to do my part to raise a generation of brilliant scientists who will find a cure for breast cancer, so that nobody else will have to go through what you're having to face.

I imagine it makes you angry sometimes, the unfairness of having to cope with cancer. As the Peeps said in the vacuum chamber, IT REALLY SUCKS. Don't forget to laugh sometimes, and I'll keep you in my thoughts. — Cathy P.

Dear friend,

Hi, I'm Juliette (and no, I have not found my romeo. I'm only 12 and people keep asking me that.) Keep pushing, and we can beat Cancer. I have a dog named cookie, a dog named snickers, a bird named Feathers, and a other bird named Peanut butter, and they wish you all the luck in the world. I go to middle school, and were are learning how to take a percent from a whole number, which I dont get. I hope you get beter, and my siblings would too, but I dont have any. Anyway, never stop dreaming. ☺

From,

Juliette.

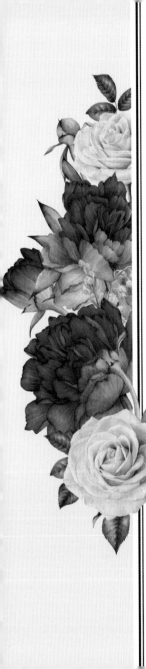

Dear Sister,

I am a 26 year survivor! I was diagnosed with Breast Cancer when I was 42 years old. I was fortunate to live in Southern California & find treatment at UCLA Medical Center. There I agreed to be part of a 5 year clinical trial study for The drug TAmoxifen (Nolvadex®) I have been Cancer free but I am always checking ✓✓ I am Thinking about you and your Treatment. I encourage you to join a group who will talk about Their health, family, health insurance and other Concerns. I found These groups to be very helpful toward my Cure — Jewell M.

DEAR GIRLFRIEND,

THIS IS A VERY FRIGHTENING TIME FOR YOU. I KNOW. I HAVE BEEN THROUGH IT, TOO. THERE IS HOPE.

KEEP SMILING. FIND THE HUMOR. WE CAN CHOOSE TO BE POSITIVE. SOME OF MY WORST MOMENTS WERE OVER SHADOWED BY HOW ABSURD AND HYSTERICAL THE NEXT MOMENT WAS.

I TOLD PEOPLE I DID NOT WANT THEIR SYMPATHY.... INSTEAD TO TELL ME A JOKE. YOU CANNOT CRY IF YOU ARE STARTING TO GIGGLE.

A SMART CHOICE I MADE AT THE BEGINNING OF MY JOURNEY WAS TO WRITE ON AN ON-LINE BLOG. ONLY MY

FRIENDS AND RELATIVES
COULD READ IT. I COULD
WRITE WHATEVER I WANTED.
MY FOLLOWERS COULD READ
ABOUT MY APPOINTMENTS,
SILLY STORIES (LIKE GETTING
STUCK IN THE HOSPITAL GARAGE
ELEVATOR WHEN THE POWER
WENT OUT.) OR WRITE ABOUT
MY FEELINGS THAT DAY. THE
PEOPLE COULD THEN LEAVE
ME A SHORT MESSAGE IF
THEY WANTED TO ENCOURAGE
ME TO "HANG IN THERE".
WITH THE BLOG I FELT NO
GUILT ABOUT NOT RETURNING
PHONE CALLS OR EMAILS.

THIS IS A JOKE I POSTED ON
MY BLOG ONE DAY.

THE DUMB BLONDE WAS
SURPRISED ONE DAY BY A
HEAVY SNOW STORM. SHE

REMEMBERED SOME ADVISE...
"FOLLOW A SNOW PLOW AND YOU
WON'T GET STUCK." LUCKY FOR
THE BLONDE SHE SAW A
SNOW PLOW AND BEGAN TO
FOLLOW. ON AND ON, THROUGH
EACH TURN SHE FOLLOWED. AT
ONE POINT THE PLOW STOPPED,
THE DRIVER GOT OUT AND
TAPPED ON THE BLONDE'S WINDOW.
"ARE YOU OK?" HE ASKED. "OH, YES,
MY DADDY ALWAYS SAID TO
FOLLOW A SNOW PLOW THROUGH
A STORM." SHE ANSWERED.
HE DIPPED HIS CAP AND SAID,
"OK, SUIT YOURSELF. I AM DONE
PLOWING THE SEAR'S PARKING
LOT AND AM GOING TO WALMART
NEXT!" KEEP SMILING!

DONNA H.

Dear Sister,
Here's a little humor from a 4-year old:

Q: Why did the banana go to the hospital?
A: Because it was not "peeling" well!

♡Love, Dawn + Caylin

Dear Friend,

I am writing to you today to wish you well, and to let you know that many People are thinking of you.

Take time to rest! When you feel tired it's okay to say - "I need a rest!" I've had treatment for Ovarian cancer and I figured out that Patience and Relaxation are very important to getting Energy Back. Try small snacks if a regular meal seems like too much. Drink lots of fluids too.

Watch Comedy shows because Laughing is what we need! It always makes me feel better to laugh and helps keep up my Spirits.

I'll be thinking of you, and best of luck - + Lots of Love from a friend - Stephanie H.

Take Your time - Feel Better!

XOX OX

Dear Friend,

My name is Miranda & I wanted to tell you of how strong & brave I think you are. I can't begin to imagine the battle you have fought up to this point, but I want to let you know you are in my thoughts. There is a horrible rumor that women are really catty to other women, but see the people who started that don't know just how connected we all are. We laugh together, we love together, and most importantly we fight battles together. So if ever there is a time when you're feeling alone, please think back to this note & know that I'm giving you all my strength. You will beat this. And then we'll all fight until we can make this horrible disease disappear. I look forward to a day that cancer becomes a memory & it is your journey that lets me know it is not a dream, but a fact. You are my hero.

XOXO,
Miranda

Fellow
Survivor

HEy sister—
Welcome to the most
elite club that you
never wanted to be invited
to. You are part of a
sisterhood that you will
have support everywhere.
I'm in Texas & consider
me one of those cheering
you onto VICTORY!! There
will be normal again, a
new normal but still life
will continue. Allison C.

my name is Bernadette, I was diagnosed with breast cancer Dec. 2005. It was a scary feeling. I went through a roller coaster of emotions. I went through chemotherapy, radiation, 5 years of hormone therapy to lower my estrogren level. I had side effects from the chemotherapy, But I made it through and am in remission. Think of chemotherapy as a healing for your body. "Cancer cannot cripple love

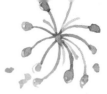

It cannot shatter hope,
It cannot corrode faith
It cannot destroy peace
It cannot kill friendship
It cannot silence courage
It cannot conquer the
spirit."
were there is A dream
there is hope, where
there is hope there is
progress, where there is
progress we gain know-
ledge to find a cure
. Take care Bernadette

Dear Friend
Hello! My name is
Sandy and I live in
Florida.
I just sat down with
my morning cup of
coffee and thought I'd
drop a note to you
with sunshine, butterflies
and wishes for a Good
Day. Butterflies are my
favorite thing.
I want you to know
you have lots of sisters
cheering for you and
sending you Hugs!
You are Special and we
all wish for Better Days for
You.
            Sandy M

Dear friend,

My name is Madison and I'm 10 years old. I'm a Girl Scout with troop 15164. I love animals and have a dog named Roxy and a cat named Shadow. Do you like animals? I'm writing to you to show my support for the journey you are on. You are so brave and I want you to know that you are not alone. My neighbor is going through this too. Sometimes my mom gets home from work and stays outside talking to her to see how she is doing. I hope you have a neighbor that checks in on you too. My wish for you is to be surrounded by people that care about you.

Sincerely,

Madison ♥

Dear Lovely Lady,
   I debated using this
sationary – although its
pretty, I found this
stationary in some
rubble after a storage
unit caught on fire
I debated using the
paper until I realized
what a metaphor it is
with you! Although the
pretty paper went
through the horrible
ordeal of a fire, fire
fighters hosing the
owners belongings, then
layed on the lawn, to dry

It remained ever
so beautiful with
so much to give —
such as, hopefully, a
smile on your face!

You will get through this
pretty lady + glow even
more with a light of
strength + courage from
inside!

Be Positive,
    Your friend,
        Courtney

Dear Friend,

I'm writing to you from Northern Kentucky on a particularly lovely ~~fall~~ evening. I wait all year for weather like this, and ~~savor~~ each swish of the crisp breeze and each rustle of fallen leaves.

As I write, I wonder if the weather chat sounds trite — which I don't want it to. I'm hoping to remind you of the light at the end of the tunnel — your own "fall weather," if you will. The challenges you face now can be overcome — and you _will_ overcome them! ~~When~~ When you do, there is so much to look forward to.

Remember, you are strong. You are courageous. You are ~~beautiful~~ beautiful, and I am sending good thoughts and hopes your way.

All my best,

Lindsay

Hello friend,

My name is Ria, and I am 11 years old. The one thing that I am absolutely sure of is that women are the strongest species alive. When something prevents us from achieving our dreams, we don't let it. When we get thrown down, we get right back up. We are built of confidence and strength.

Three years ago, my parents got divorced. I remember feeling devasted, like I couldn't get back up. It was at this point time when I reminded myself that no matter how many clouds cover the sky, the sunshine always peeks out. My attitude turned things around for me. You are a warrior, too. I wrote the poem below to tell the story of a beautiful, strong woman, just like you.

Her eyes, whom have beared many tears
Her face, that has challenged many fears
Her story, that has brightened many days
Her soul, as strong as sun's rays
Her body, that has empowered through a lot
Her strength, that has loved and fought
Her heart, which has given me hope
Her life, which has had so much to cope
Her mind, gleaming with rhyme and reason
Her smile, getting brighter with each season
Her attitude, so ready to experience life as it comes

Lots of Love,
Ria ♡ ♡ ♡ ♡

Dear friend,

Greetings! I hope today has been a good day and that tomorrow will be even better. I know that you will be able to cope with the challenges that come — have faith in yourself, that you are strong enough to fight, and remember that we are all with you, thinking about you, and willing to do what we can to help you get through.

I'm writing to you from Botswana, in Southern Africa. I'm here working with an organization working to set up cervical cancer prevention + care programs. Screening and treatment are badly needed, and when they are available, I remember how much we are all the same — women everywhere, trying to be strong and keep

ourselves healthy so we can be there
to take care of the people we love. The
women who come for services don't always
speak English, and I don't know
much about their lives, or what they
hope for, or what their stories are.
But strength and kindness are universal,
and if I can't talk to them, at least
I can talk to you, since we are all sisters
in a way and need to look out for each
other. You are in good company - there
are so many who would share their
stories, their strength and their love
with you.

      With warmest wishes,

          Alisha

Dearest Lady —

Let me tell you about a medium of the 1940's. She ran the Happy Bottom Riding Ranch or what is now Edwards Airforce, Poncho, as I knew, here was a Brevet (career Survivor). She never wore "fake boots". Just flannel shirt, Kackie Pants & cowboy boots. She was to be honored at a reunion on Edward AFB with a lot of other pilots (she flew with Amelia Earheart) (Barnstormed & flew for the movies) One day we were trying planes & flew for the movies) One day we met at the post office — She ask me to pad her special dress (Blue Sequins) so she had boots — I did — She kept saying Bigger — Her Blackwig, So the night come — Her Blackwig, Big Boots & Blue Sequins was not what stood out that night — What glittered & shown was a fighter, a lady who played by her rules & forgot

Cancer — She did not let it win. So dear lovely — When you have a down day — google Poncho Barn's — She i+ was a Great Counter + lovely i) the Mojave desert, + I was lucky to call her My friend! She dared to be different.

Take Care + know you one in my thoughts!

Hugs
Irene R.

Dear Friend,

My name is Jenna. I am a thirteen year old girl. I am writing this letter from the hospital, where I have come to recover from my own illness. I may not know exactly what it is that you are going through, and I may not ever. But I understand myself and what I have gone through. At times you are going to feel as if there is no point anymore, as if it has never been harder to pick yourself up and do all you can for yourself. I am not going to tell you to ignore these feelings. Instead, I wish for you to remember them always and allow them to be your reason to carry on, and to work even harder. I failed to do that at many times in my life, I allowed them to push me in the wrong direction and I thought it would be more than impossible to turn it all around. I can honestly say that at one point, I wanted nothing more than for my life to end. Then one morning I woke up and looked out my window to see a beautiful sunrise. I almost took that privilege away from myself forever. The one thing I wish I could share with everyone, is to never ever miss out on anything you want to do. If something really makes you happy, forget all the risks, don't overthink it. Just hold on to it forever.

Honestly, life is much, much too short to be
scared or unhappy or angry at time and
circumstances. Do not try to avoid
them. Let them happen. Life is sad, but oh is
it beautiful. You are a beautiful piece of a
beautiful world, so don't ever treat yourself like
you are anything less. A month ago, I had no idea
what my purpose is. Now? I am positive that my
purpose is to inform people like you that your life
is valuable. So contribute valuable things.
    Best wishes for you, and take care.
      Jenna

Dear friend,

We may not have met, but I know you are strong. You are a fighter. You can+ will beat this. I will be thinking of you as you go thru your battle and come out on top. Let me hear your battlecry!!

Jessica

Dear sister,

you might not be aware of this, but women all over the world are thinking about you right now. we are sending you strength and positivity. we are there with you, right now, holding your hand.

we don't know each other personally, but it does not matter. your fight is our fight. your pain is our pain. And together, we will get through anything. I am 30 years old but still have much learning to do to become the woman I want to be. your courage gives me the confidence to know that women can face any challenge head on and win. The circle of inspiration that flows from woman to woman, over barriers" like race, creed or economic status, will continue to be strong and unbreakable- thanks to amazing women like you! we are all here for you and we all love you.

I offer to you my unending support and I think of you daily. we'll never meet, but that does not mean I will stop sending positivity to every corner of this world, knowing that it will reach you and other women. Do not give up your fight! you are not alone. you are important. most of all, you are loved.

with encouragement,
Jasmin

DEAR FRIEND,

You don't know my twin sister but I'll bet you know people like her. She's funny, quick-thinking, and always the one ready to help anyone in need. So when she was diagnosed with breast cancer, I wanted to know why her. Why does such a good person get sick? You may be asking yourself the same

question. I still don't know the answer.

What I do know is that my sister never cried, at least not in front of the family. She opted for additional genetic testing to be sure as her twin I was okay. Every day after radiation treatments she ate Cheetos and didn't care about fat thighs or orange stains. When the doctor told her she was cancer-free, she took a trip to Russia because she'd never been. And when she told me how much she loved me and the family and threw her arms around me, I knew she was changed forever.

There are so many questions we can't answer, but I know you will soon wrap your arms around your loved ones as a cancer-free survivor. My twin sister has never asked why her. She told me - "If I ask why for the bad stuff, then I have to ask why for the good stuff too." I think she's right. But I also think it's fair and human to think about it. I hope you can take this time to give yourself a break. EAt

Cheetos and do whatever makes you happy. My sister used cancer as a seperation from her normal life and gave herself time to heal. I hope you do the same.

From all the sisters in the world, both actual and in spirit, I wish you a speedy recovery and wonderful future. I know 1 in 8 women get breast cancer, so I guess this time you're taking one for the team. Thank you!

Your sister, Sara H.

Dear Brave Woman—

Yes. You are brave. You may also be scared, but above all things— You are brave! Remember that. Keep fighting. Fight for the people you love to wrap your arms around. Fight for all the younger women whom you inspire. Fight for women everywhere so we can one day tell our children + grandchildren that Breast Cancer is 100% treatable + recoverable. Fight to read your favorite book, eat your favorite meal, visit your favorite place again + again + again. You are so strong. You can beat this. You will triumph. Keep fighting!

XOXO XO

Heidi

Hello Sister,

I am a 2 year breast cancer survivor

the Positive thought for the day —

When you feel no one cares or loves you, everyone is ignoring you, and people are jealous of you, ask yourself

Am I Just Too Sexy?

Keep Smiling
Judy

Dear Sister,

When you hurt, those around you hurt. I learned how much twenty years ago.

I remember, like it was yesterday, the sinking feeling when I saw the nurse in the hall point to my room and say the results weren't good.

My strength came from friends and loved ones and a doctor who never gave up on me. <u>Now I celebrate</u> CELEBRATE your anniversaries — 1 year, 5 years, 10 years — Yes! 20 years celebrate who you are. You are stronger than you think. You mean so much to so many. Be proud of who you are. Hold your head high and "go for the ~~gold~~ pink."

Believe + Achieve
In Sisterly Love,
Karen V.

Dear Friend,

The other day I took my dog Coda to the dog park and he peed on a lady's skirt. They don't make a card for that! Here's wishing you good health and a dry skirt.

Hoping you laugh,

Grant

Stay Strong,
One day
at a time.
You will get there.
Take care.

Dear friend,

    You are a great woman. You know how I know that without ever meeting you? You are a fighter and stronger than anything life can throw at you, and as a woman you can endure it all with grace, beauty, and a sense of humor. I know you are great because as women we all are, but women like you are even more special. I'm truly inspired by women like you who receive news that shakes up their life, but press on. I'll say it again...you're a fighter ☺ Even though my greatest hope is that we can look back and say "remember when cancer existed?" Until that day it's women like you who give those around you hope & strength. Thank you! So, love, laugh, and spend each moment doing what makes you willdly happy because that should be all of our goals! Sincerly & with love & awe,

                          Sara

Sister,

We don't know each other but I must say you are one of many people whom I look up to. Isn't it amazing that you have no idea who I am, or what I'm like ... But, somehow you encourage and inspire me in such a way? Somehow you manage to help me believe that anything is possible if you have strength, faith, and courage. I never thought I'd get the opportunity to write such a strong individual, like yourself, to thank you for being such a great inspiration. You've taught me that you don't need fists to fight, but fighting like a girl is easier because you just need a warm, strong heart. Wow! It's so much I want to say, but words couldn't even explain my thoughts. People everywhere go through many things and face plenty of obstacles, but yours indeed is very important. You've won your battle in the ring and the fighting was worth it. A special, strong **survivor** is what I'd call you. I've never been placed in a situation such as this, but just from hearing your story, I believe I am prepared and have the tools ready to become a survivor. From me to you, I would like to say keep fighting, be strong, continue to believe in yourself and you will continue to encourage young females like you and myself.

Love,
Alexis

Dear Friend,

"Laughter is great medicine," my mom liked to say. And my mother had a funny bone. We were shopping one day when a woman with a particularly long nose walked by. Mom stopped and did a double take. "Nose, where are you going with that woman," she stated with conviction. We all fell over laughing! It struck us so funny—that line is now part of our family sayings. Like Grandma used to say about Grandpa's old fashioned ideas— "If he could, he'd park a horse and buggy in the garage."

Sending you a smile from my heart to make your day a little lighter.   Iris

Dear Sister,

The time when I was overwhelmed with the pain and emotionality of what was happening to me I was shown my next step by listening to the deepest of my cries. Perhaps this is somewhat like what you are feeling as a diagnosis brings many painful assessments of ambiguities and all these who, and why and when. It's enough to make you dizzy at times— and even confused.

I hope you can find the courage to wade through the dizzy and confusion and get to your deepest cry - the one that echoes that your very soul feels like it is sinking and drowning out of the reach of the feel of life. Because in this lie 2 important questions to ask yourself to regain your footing & your focus: How do I regain my wonder at being alive? and what must I do to keep my heart from sinking?

Know that there is a drive in each of our heart's capacity to rise up - no matter how bruised we feel, that verifies we have the power in as to face things head on. AND to move our whole being through- Take heart - there are many women like me rooting + cheering you on. Be gentle with yourself.

Sincerely, Connie

Dear sister,♡

My name is Mattie, I can not imagine what you are going through rite now. But I am here to say you are strong and keep your head-up. You are an amazing person and you will get through this struggle. Before you know it you will be 100% and having the time of your life. So, whenever you feel alone know that it will be better soon& you will always be on my mind. When I was 10 my Grandma Karla was diagnosed with breast cancer and within 3 years she was 100%, running around and playing with me again. It all happened so fast it was almost as if it never happened. So, don't worry it will all be over soon. ☺ And Remember you are very strong and also my hero.

love Always,
♡Mattie

Never give up!

To an amazing woman!
From the netherlands, J want
you to know, that someone
cares. My sister got breastcancer,
41 years young. J do remember her first
words; " J m walking on eggshells ", when
she came from the specialist. But her next words were; " J will win!!"
J want you to say; You're important!
Take one step at a time! And J
want you to know that someone cares
about you! Yes; really, even in the
Netherlands! My goal, give love 8
power to you!

Hugs 8 Love
Jette S.

There's a 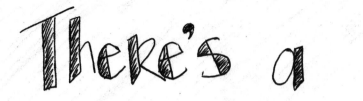 REASON...

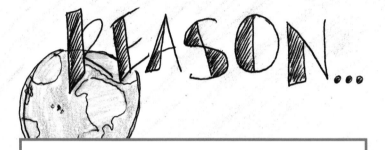

the world's still turning: it's for you
to have another day to fight, grow, & win!
Keep fighting, you can beat this!
Thank you for the example of strength
& endurance you are to me &
everyone else whose life you touch!
The hearts of so many people are
rooting for you!
Love,
Caitlin

Dear friend,

My name is Abbey. I live way out in the middle of no where and don't know that much about breast cancer. I know it's a hard thing to go through, though. I also know you're stronger than cancer and can beat this. You may not have ever heard of a show called George Lopez, but everytime he faces a challenge he screams, "I GOT THIS!" That's what I want you to do from here on out. Feeling down and out? You scream I got this! and that way you'll remember how strong you are and how you'll get through this. I hope you also rememblr all the strangers out there — like my self — that are rooting for you. We know you can do it girl! Hang in there!

I drew a monkey "hanging in there" to show you my awesome art skills

monkey

Sincerely,
Abbey J., 10th grade

P.S. — I'm an awful speller. Please excuse all my mistakes.

Dear friend -
A poem I wrote for you.

WISHING YOU PEACE TODAY

I am sending you this greeting -
   a smile also -
      your way -
If you are hurting or in pain Anywhere -
weather it be in body or mind -
I am sending you Peace -
to let you know -
   everything is going to be fine.

I know that this storm is raging–
and it may be tearing at your sails–
just wanted you to know–
   Peace is gonna prevail.
We all have our own boat–in the sea
   called Life– hold on– do what you
can– let others help you– when it's
hard to stand– We are with you–
to help you fight this beast–
You are already the winner.
AND I SEND YOU PEACE.

Thinking of
you!
Heather
!!

Dear Friend,

May the light always find you on a dreary day. When you need to be home, may you find your way. May you always have courage to take a chance. And never find frogs in your underpants.

— An Irish toast

Continue to laugh!

You are strong!
You are fabulous!
You are powerful!

Sincerely,
Perry W.

Dear Friend,

My thoughts are with you as you go through your unexpected journey. May the love and kindness of family and friends, and caring strangers, help you through.

Sometimes what we are looking for is right in front of us and we can't see it. Recently, my friend Susan and I were meeting for dinner at a Thai restaurant. We ended up waiting nearly half an hour for each other. Turns out we were both waiting in the restaurant at separate tables. Thank goodness for cell phones.

Be strong and may you find what you are looking for and get the healing you need.

Best wishes for peace, love and healing,
Margie W.

Dear Friend,

I know you are concerned having recently been diagnosed with breast cancer. But, I want to

encourage you with the fact that I have friends who have come through the diagnosis & treatment with great success. In fact, I have one friend who had a Stage 4 diagnosis, and she has been doing great, and she was diagnosed 14 years ago. She works with a lot of little children in special classes in school.

So, take courage, think positively, and know that all your friends, both known and unknown, are pulling for you!

Sincerely,
Nola

Dear Sister,

I went to hear an inspirational speaker talk and I learned something interesting about carpentry. When two beams support a joist on either side of it, it's called "SISTERING." Isn't that wonderful? Such a cool term. Because that's what women do— we hold each other up. So no matter where you are, imagine yourself being held up and supported by a sister in IL who is rooting for you!

♡Love,
Dawn

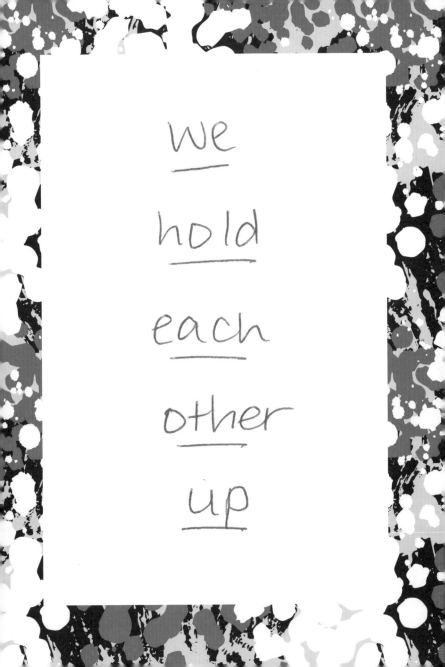

Dear Sister,

I am a scientist, and have spent my entire career dedicated to the pursuit of new drug discovery. What motivates me in my job is the needs of patients, and how their lives could be improved. Although I do not know you, I am thinking of you, and what your experience might be. I think of you as a daughter, a mother, a sister or a friend. I know that you are not

...defined by your diagnosis, and I wish you the best in your treatment and recovery. Please know that each caregiver, and behind every medicine is someone who cares about you and your well-being. My colleagues and I are never satisfied with existing treatment realities, and we are working hard to provide ever-improving options to improve patient reality.

Sincerely,
Ted.

Dear Friend,

A wise, beautiful soul once told me that the greatest gift you can give to someone is the opportunity to give to you. The truth of these words became more & more evident as I supported & cared for her throughout her battle with breast cancer. Her grace, courage & unwavering sense of hope inspired & humbled me. I encourage you to reach out to those around you & to allow them to care for ~~them~~ you during this time as you focus on your healing. May you find peace & joy in each passing day. Love, Whitney

Greetings!

In a few weeks, we will celebrate my Aunt's 90th birthday! She is a botanist, an adventurer, a world traveler, a teacher, a mother & grandmother & my much loved Aunt. She is also a survivor of a double mastectomy which she had 45 years ago. She has always been an inspiration to me! There are so many of us sending you good thoughts for this fight!

Cynthia H.

Dear Friend,

As I look back over the years, Especially the last forty-six years, I see so many changes in my life. First and foremost almost that long ago. It was in July 25th that I got married. It's hard to believe, I don't really feel that old. I'm I am now seventy-one and my husband is I am now eighty-two. He is still very active, always doing something. Years ago he went to a regular job. Now that he is retired, he gardens, builds things, even works on our vehicles.

You might ask, what do I do? Years ago I worked in an office. Now I still do office work at home. Besides the general bookkeeping, I'm the chief cook and dishwasher. When ree things in Radicchen unions and prepare it sitting for a meal n storage in the refrigerator. We also have Swiss chard from the garden and even corn growing. Plus a variety of different kinds of beans.

Other than bookkeeping, housework and writing, things I enjoy reading and sewing to.

Sincerely,

On occasions I get a chance to go to a movie, besides the regular grocery shopping. Even a few errands for my husband. So he requests items from Home Depot or Sams or for plumbing parts.

Whichever and whenever, I'm needed and dependant upon. Just as you are to maintain your health and well being.

How are you doing? How is your family? I hope they are there to hold your hand or give you an encouraging word or two ... Besides "I love you".

If not... take my advice, help yourself feel better. Try in that dream, you've been meaning to buy on.

Or read something different. Like a cook book or history. Walk out into the sunshine and enjoy the beauty of the day.

If you're a night person, go outside and look up at the stars. Revel in the beauty of yourself and motivate. You're beautiful because you are special and also a friend, so you listen to your own body. It tells you, when you are thirsty, hungry or even in some pain. Don't ignore it!

There is always someone that will listen to you... If not, start a diary or a letter to yourself.

always in friendship,
Lynn

Dear Sister ♡

Words cannot truly convey
how much I wish I was there
with you now to help you cope with this
disease. Know this, my spirit and thoughts are
with you, holding your hand through it all. You have
a hard journey ahead of you, but I know you can
do it. I know you can stand triumphant at the end
of your journey. You are STRONG. Always remember that.

Albert Camus once said, "In the depth of winter, I finally
learned that within me there lay an invincible summer."
You have that summer, that strength, inside of you and it will
help you get through this. You are a fighter. I cannot begin to
understand what you are going through right now as I am only 14
and have not experienced your fears before. But I do know that
everyone is capable of overcoming hardship. And that it is in those
struggles that we truly discover who we are. You are a beautiful,
amazing, POWERFUL woman. And you can do anything.

During all of your treatment, please remember that there are
hundreds of people cheering you on and willing you to succeed. No matter
how much it feels like it, you are NOT alone. The thoughts and hopes
of women across the world are with you always.

Also, NEVER EVER GIVE UP HOPE. You will make it through this. And while life might never be the same, you will emerge from your fight stronger and more confident in your self as a woman. You will see that you can accomplish anything because you are a fighter and a believer. More than anything, I hope that during your battle you feel loved. I hope you realize and feel the messages of warmth and care that are being sent to you every moment of every day. I hope you understand and the love that everyone feels for you and how strongly everyone is rooting for you!

So hold you head up because you WILL make it through. No matter what, keep fighting.

I am sending love to you
ALWAYS~

♡ Kaitlyn C.

Hello my friend,

Wouldn't it be fun to just sit on a blanket in a shady grove and watch the birds and butterflies come and go? And after a while, you could pick the fruit you love best and savor the juices and pulp of your choice! It could be a time to escape your worries, concerns, pain... Your imagination is alive and well — don't let the cancer take that away from you! Go on a "mind trip" every day to your favorite places, whether land, sea or air. Fly like an eagle and escape that body for awhile! That's what I do when I'm homebound and in pain. It gives me joy to let my mind and senses soar — no longer bound by body restrictions. I hope you will give it a try! It might be the best trip you've ever taken! I'll see you in the clouds!

Hugs to you, Susan

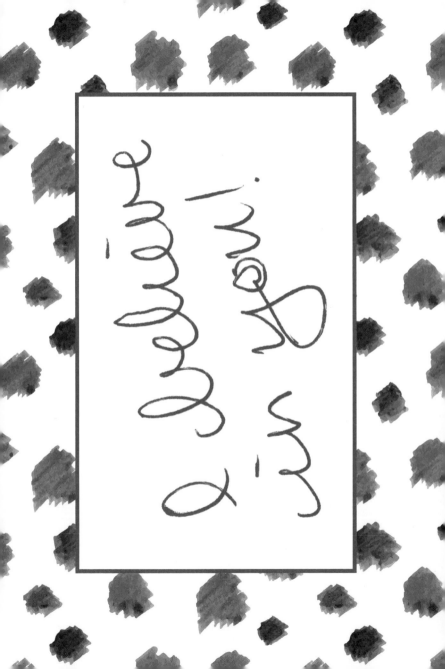

Dear Fighter,
My name is Elijah, I am 11 years old.
I was born in America and I
immigrated to Haifa, Israel. When my
grandma was 32 she had breast cancer
and now she is 60 and still active and fun!
Keep on fighting. Don't give up!
Here are some jokes to make you laugh:

What is brown and   sticky?
a stick

What is the best air?
millionaire

from
Elijah

Dear Sister,

I was in your shoes five months ago, and I would like to tell you that you are braver and stronger than you ever thought you could be! It's okay to be scared, angry and confused, but hope, love and courage will get you through this journey. You're not alone. You are strong, you are while. You are beautiful. You are while.

Love, Susan P.

"A girl should be two things classy and Fabulous"
— Coco Chanel

"A woman has to live her life, or live to repent not
having lived it" — DH Lawrence, Lady Chatterly's Lover

Dear friend,

Now is a trying time I am sure. I know
you can think of and endless number of
things you would rather be doing than
undertaking the battle you are about to fight
But now is not the time to dwell on the
negative, but praise and rejoice in the positive.

You are a woman!!! An endless enigma
of splendor and mystery, we women have
kept things turning, kept people motivated
and loved throughout the ages. Go outside
and yell to the sky "I am a women,
here me and know I am the most fierce
creature ever created!"

Now is the time to take down that list.
Write everything down you have ever wanted
to accomplish. It's your fight list! These are
your personalized and tailored moves to beat
your opponet because you will beat it.
The odds are in your favor because you are
a woman and you have so many secret
weapons.
Faith... Compassion... Courage... Anger!

Maybe you are used to it but if not step outside of that comfort zone. Read Lady Chatterly's Lover, go to a movie by yourself, go buy yourself the most beautiful flowers you can find.

All of these are arrows in your quiver that will quell this sickness and after you beat it I want to see a victory dance. Like a flash mob victory dance. Big Bold Brilliant!

You are a woman. My sister, my friend if I was ever fortunate enough to cross your path, I salute you an applaud you. I believe in you, in your strength.

So if you haven't already fall in love, with someone or something! fret in trouble... with someone or something ☺ Fly, cry, carress and undress! Buy something outrageous and reach out with kindness that is only from the storybooks. Live, hate, envy, and feel supreme. Because you are a women, a symbol of strength and of endless change

Be strong my friend
Neale C.

Hello Friend.

On This very hot day I do like to sit for awhile + have a cup of tea join me if you can. My house is cool. My son makes sure he keeps it that way for me. I live with him + his wife. I had to move from my home I couldn't stay by myself. It is better than an "old ladies" home. I have my own apartment. I am much happier as I'll say bye for now.

Your friend
Apartment

Dear Friend,

No one knows exactly what you are going through but I hope you can find comfort in the efforts as we try to understand. We're going to get it wrong sometimes, overstep our bounds, get in the way, but we can't stop trying. We want you better!

Mary L.

Dear Friend,

I'm sure you're already hearing all the time, "I can't imagine what you're going through." But really, a lot of us can. We imagine it all the time. We've had mammograms and mammogram callbacks and ultrasounds and MRI's and biopsies, and we've endured the excruciating wait for the doctor to call. And many have gotten the news that you have, that there's more to do.

I can imagine what you're going through because I've had some experience with it, too—the lump, the mammogram, the ultrasound, the callback, another mammogram, a sit-down with the radiologist in front of a blue screen in an ice-cold office. Then a biopsy and the wait for the phone call. Every step of the way, my fears ballooned and took my imagination into corners where it didn't belong.

I'm a writer/reporter by profession, and I wanted to know as much as I possibly could about my situation, the treatment options, the statistics, the outcomes. I didn't want platitudes about how everything would be okay. I wanted real information and solid answers. The medical pros by my side were warm and experienced, and they answered all my questions about what might come next, and they carefully explained the reasons why (they also gave me excellent advice that I will pass along: Stay off the Internet! Dr. Google is not your friend right now.)

My takeaway? The breast cancer detection and treatment industry is finely tuned and well-oiled, and this is a _great_ thing. Research has taught our medical pros so much, and we can overcome this disease. This is one area of medicine where they've really got it together. Between my fears and frustrations, I was able to be very grateful we've come so far.

You will benefit from that. You've got "sisters" everywhere who have been there, who have come out the other side healthy and strong, and you will, too. It's modern medicine at its finest—and that, my friend, will help assure you, even when you might feel stuck in those dark corners of your imagination, that everything really will be okay.

Sincerely,
Krista M.

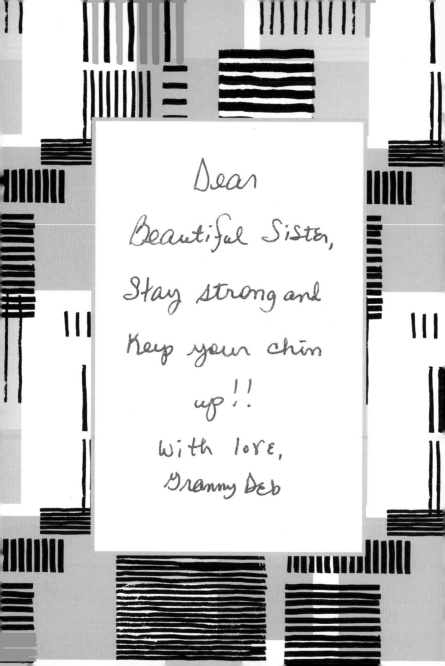

Dear
Beautiful Sister,
Stay strong and
Keep your chin
up!!
With love,
Granny Deb

Dear Friend,

Hello there! Today I did my daily run and I offered it up for you. With each step I focused on sending healing thoughts your way! Times are tough for you right now, but they won't always be this way. You are strong, courageous and so very loved. Your friends and family are pulling for you and wishing for a speedy recovery.

H old On! Pain Ends. (hope)

You can do this just one day at a time. Brighter tomorrows are ahead!

Love,
☺ Martha

Dear Sister,

My housemate Linda (I call her "Goddess of Happiness") has two black cats. Well, Mocha, she's all black, with a round face that seems to say "I'm older than I look." Gracie has a white heart-shape patch on her chest.

Mocha had me trained by Week Two. I would be in my room, writing. I hear a meow. I open my door. There she is, looking up at me. Then she starts down the stairs and stops at the front door. Oh, I get it. We leave. I return to my work.

An hour later, I hear a meow. It takes me one whole minute to realize that was Mocha's "signal." I'm back. "You need to come down and open the front door for me."

Sorry, Mocha, I'll be quicker next time.
Little Gracie does not meow when she wants to go out,
she stands near the front door and waits for a human to
notice her. When she wants to come in she knocks. I am not
kidding. I wish there was a peep hole twelve inches from
the ground so that we can see thou the door this with
her head? With her hip?

Mocha and Gracie have distinctive ways to ask for —
what they need, what they want. This is what I wish I with
you — that you, Goddess of Bravery, will
always get what you need, (what you want.

From very caring people —
I send you gentle hugs.

Sincerely,
Teresa L.

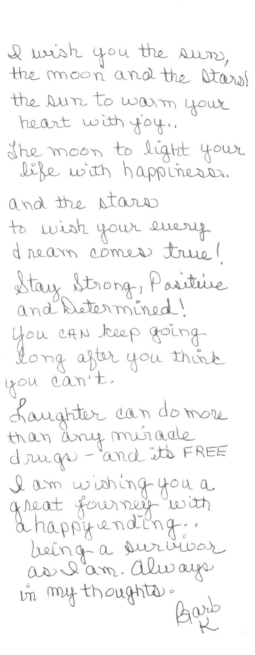

I wish you the sun,
the moon and the Stars!
the sun to warm your
 heart with joy..
The moon to light your
 life with happiness..

and the stars
to wish your every
dream comes true!

Stay Strong, Positive
and Determined!
You CAN keep going
long after you think
you can't.

Laughter can do more
than any miracle
drugs — and its FREE

I am wishing you a
great journey with
a happy ending..
 being a survivor
as I am. Always
in my thoughts.

Barb
K

Dearest Friend,

My name is Kaori and I have been cancer free for over three years!

When I was diagnosed, I was simply shocked. I have been living very healthy life style, daily exercise, yoga, eating right, everything that should have prevented from me getting any kind of diseases, especially cancer. But I got it, so I took cancer as an opportunity to take a closer look at my own life.

During the whole process (tests surgeries, and radiation), I have learned how fragile I was and at the same time, how strong I could be. Over all, it might be strange statement to make but cancer made me a better person, because I accepted who I was.

You might be going through the "why" phase, asking what caused cancer, but in the end, its does not matter how you got here. The most important thing is where can you go from here. Wherever you are, I am writing to you to let you know you are not alone with this journey!

lots of love K

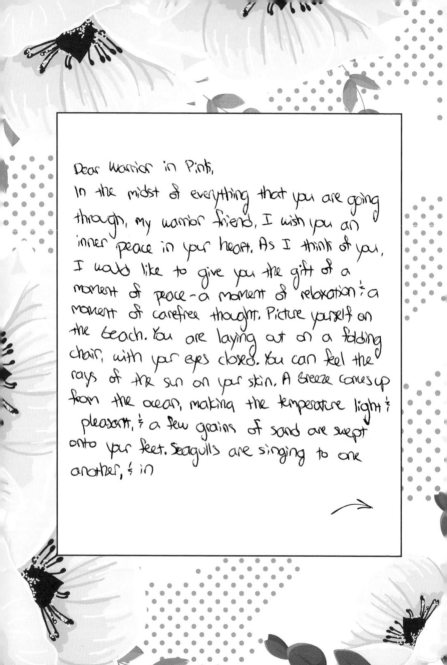

Dear Warrior in Pink,

In the midst of everything that you are going through, my warrior friend, I wish you an inner peace in your heart. As I think of you, I would like to give you the gift of a moment of peace - a moment of relaxation ÷ a moment of carefree thought. Picture yourself on the beach. You are laying out on a folding chair, with your eyes closed. You can feel the rays of the sun on your skin. A breeze comes up from the ocean, making the temperature light ÷ pleasant, ÷ a few grains of sand are swept onto your feet. Seagulls are singing to one another, ÷ in the distance, you hear the sound of young children laughing together & splashing in the ocean waves. The waves crash gently upon the shore, in a rhythmic & repetitive movement. For just a moment, stay & linger in this world, at this beach. Breathe deeply & enjoy this moment of peace. Give yourself this gift. Whenever you need a moment of peace, take it for yourself & allow yourself this small indulgence. I am thinking of you & wishing you peace in your heart amid the hardships & challenges of life. At the end of the day, peace always triumphs!

Thinking warmly of you & sending you much love, hope, peace, & joy!

                           - Camilla

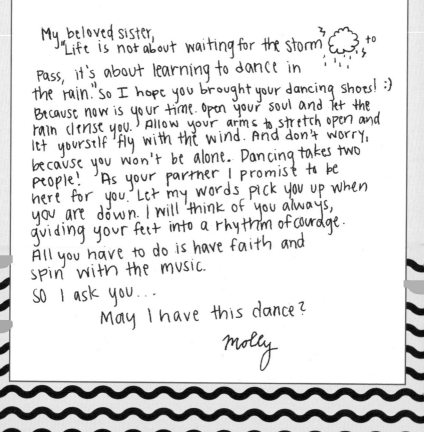

My beloved sister,
    "Life is not about waiting for the storm to Pass, it's about learning to dance in the rain." So I hope you brought your dancing shoes! :) Because now is your time. Open your soul and let the rain clense you. Allow your arms to stretch open and let yourself fly with the wind. And don't worry, because you won't be alone. Dancing takes two people! As your partner I promise to be here for you. Let my words pick you up when you are down. I will think of you always, guiding your feet into a rhythm of courage.
All you have to do is have faith and spin with the music.
So I ask you...
        May I have this dance?
                    molly

Dear Friend,
Hi, My name is Jordan. I
am 9½ years old. I'm a
boy. I'm in 4th grade
I am writing this
because I want to
make you feel better.
At our school we have
a "Go Pink!" day last friday.
We are competing with
Spanish Springs EL.

Every time I feel
Depresed I think of
a sauirrl lifting heights
Hope you get well soon
soon!
                    your friend,
                    Jordan

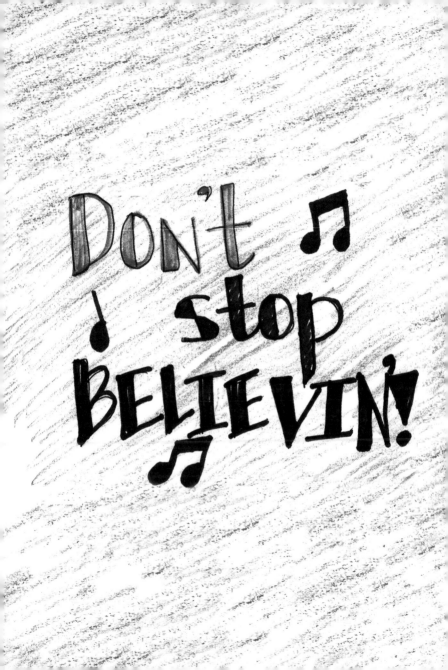

Dear Friend,

My grandmother was named Elizabeth but everyone called her Bunkie. She was a breast cancer survivor. She was also an amazing cook, an avid gardener, and loved the Blue Ridge Mountains. So many of my best memories are from summers with her— going to the library, picking green beans in the garden, and watching Anne of Green Gables. She was a breast cancer survivor. I don't know you but I know there are people in your life who treasure time spent with you. Fight for them, fight for you. Women everywhere are standing behind you and standing with you.

yours,
Meg B.

ACKNOWLEDGMENTS

My Thanks to

Rachel Hiles and Deanne Katz, and the design team at
Chronicle Books for their hard work and creativity.
A special thank-you to the breast cancer centers across the
country who hand out the Girls Love Mail letters and to
the numerous organizations who support Girls Love Mail.
Girls Love Mail couldn't function without tremendous
effort from our amazing team of volunteers and our board
of directors. And, of course, our immense gratitude goes
out to all of the letter writers, both in and out of these
pages. Because of you, as of the printing of this book,
Girls Love Mail has given out over 100,000 letters; that's
over 100,000 women encouraged.

TO LEARN HOW YOU CAN HELP,
PLEASE VISIT

GirlsLoveMail.com